U0311374

世界卫生组织

降低烟草致瘾性措施咨询报告

主　译　胡清源
副主译　侯宏卫　陈　欢

科学出版社

北京

内 容 简 介

　　世界卫生组织六大区域的专家讨论了关于降低烟草致瘾性的已有和最新知识，并审查了对个人和社会可能产生的积极和消极后果，以及措施成功实施的条件和挑战，在此基础上形成了本报告。首先研究了烟碱降低措施对吸烟者和非吸烟者的潜在影响，其次探讨了烟碱降低策略对烟草控制的假定社会后果，最后总结了实施降低烟草致瘾性措施的九个方面的潜在挑战，以便决策者能够以结构化的方式了解这一策略的优点。

　　本书会引起吸烟与健康、烟草化学和公共卫生学等诸多领域研究人员的兴趣，可以为涉足烟草科学研究的科技工作者和烟草管制研究的决策者提供权威性参考，对烟草企业的生产实践也有重要的指导作用。

图书在版编目(CIP)数据

降低烟草致瘾性措施咨询报告/世界卫生组织编; 胡清源主译. —北京: 科学出版社，2019.3
书名原文: Consultation on Tobacco Addictiveness Reduction Measures
ISBN 978-7-03-060803-1

Ⅰ.①降… Ⅱ.①世… ②胡… Ⅲ.①烟草–控制–研究报告–世界 Ⅳ.①R163

中国版本图书馆CIP数据核字(2019)第044293号

责任编辑：刘　冉／责任校对：杜子昂
责任印制：吴兆东／封面设计：时代世启

科 学 出 版 社 出版
北京东黄城根北街 16 号
邮政编码：100717
http://www.sciencep.com

北京中石油彩色印刷有限责任公司 印刷
科学出版社发行　各地新华书店经销
*
2019年3月第　一　版　　开本：890×1240 A5
2019年3月第一次印刷　　印张：3
字数：90 000
定价：80.00元
（如有印装质量问题，我社负责调换）

REPORT

Consultation on Tobacco Addictiveness Reduction Measures

Berlin, Germany
15-16 May 2018

翻译委员会

主　译：胡清源

副主译：侯宏卫　陈　欢

译　者：胡清源　侯宏卫　陈　欢

　　　　张小涛　刘　彤　韩书磊

　　　　付亚宁　王红娟

目录

Contents

致 谢

感谢所有参与协商（见附录 1）并通过准备背景文件促进本报告编制的人。

Ranti Fayokun 博士在 Vinayak Prasad 博士的指导下协调了研讨过程、背景文件的编制和 WHO 报告的编写。Anastasia Vernikou 女士在 Ranti Fayokun 博士的支持下起草了本报告。Armando Peruga 教授协助完成了报告的定稿。Nicky Nicksic 博士和 Sarah Galbraith 女士总结了背景文件。Carmen Audera Lopez 博士在 Vera Luiza da Costa e Silva 博士的指导下领导并协调了世界卫生组织《烟草控制框架公约》秘书处的磋商进程。

感谢 Elie Akl 教授、Hristo Bozukov 教授、Katja Bromen 博士、Nuan Ping Cheah 博士、Denis Choiniere 先生、Priyanka Dahiya 女士、Matus Ferech 博士、Becky Freeman 博士、Marcia M Sebrao Fernandes 女士、Rishi Gupta 博士、Dorcas Kiptui 女士、Wasim Maziak 教授、Benn McGrady 博士、Andre Luiz Oliveira da Silva 先生、Moira Sy 女士、Tibor Szilagyi 博士和 Ghazi Zaatari 博士的贡献。Miriamjoy Aryee Quansah 女士提供了行政支持。

此外，还要感谢德国政府主办了此次研讨会并提供财政、技术和行政支持，感谢加拿大政府提供财政资助。

摘　要

　　应世界卫生组织《烟草控制框架公约》（WHO FCTC）缔约方会议的要求，于 2018 年 5 月在德国柏林举行了关于降低烟草致瘾性措施的会议。

　　世界卫生组织所有区域的专家讨论了关于降低烟草致瘾性的已有和最新知识，并审查了对个人和社会可能产生的积极和消极后果，以及措施成功实施的条件和挑战。尽管与会者没有就降低烟碱或烟草致瘾性政策的优缺点达成共识，但讨论的重点是充分知情辩论所需的要素，特别是燃烧型烟草制品，因为有更多证据可供利用。

　　首先，研究了烟碱降低措施对吸烟者和非吸烟者的潜在个人影响。专家认为对吸烟者的影响包括减少烟草制品的消费和寻找烟碱的替代来源。然而，对于非吸烟者而言，这些影响一方面涉及开始使用或持续使用烟草制品的可能性降低，而另一方面，基于对降低健康风险的误解，这可能会导致新手开始吸烟的可能性增加。

　　此外，专家们还探讨了烟碱降低策略对烟草控制的假定社会后果。这种方法可能会引起期望的吸烟非规范化从而使得当地或全球的吸烟减少，会减少燃烧型烟草制品的使用从而带来环境效益，会减少烟草相关疾病支出从而带来经济效益，这将具有改善卫生系统的效果。相反，烟草管制的负面社会后果可能涉及烟草制品非法贸易的增加，可能导致更高的初吸率、戒烟的减少和既往吸烟者因低价产品与非法贸易的竞争以及其他破坏烟草控制的因素而导致的复发率增加。此外，可能会影响税收，这对于政府可能是个问题。

一些专家指出，由于缺乏烟碱降低策略将减少吸烟率的普遍共识，任何讨论成功实施的条件都为时过早。然而，人们认识到，希望通过降低烟碱含量来降低烟草致瘾性的国家应考虑到政策的影响，这将取决于国家的监管背景。目前，这只适合于拥有先进、全面控制措施和广泛资源及知识以确保充分实施的国家。作为一项基本先决条件，与会者注意到确保执行世界卫生组织《烟草控制框架公约》中关键的减少需求措施的重要性，如 WHO FCTC 第 6 条、第 8 条、第 11 条、第 13 条和第 14 条及其缔约方会议通过纳入的实施指南内容。此外，强制将烟碱降低至极低致瘾性水平必须是全面烟草控制方法的一部分，该方法成功实施了关键的减少需求措施，并已建立了市场监督和产品检测能力。专家们一致认为，在对于制定指导方针有价值的国家经验出现之前，目前不适宜制定有关降低烟碱政策的指导方针。

最后，专家们总结了实施降低烟草致瘾性措施的九个方面的潜在挑战，以便决策者能够以结构化的方式了解这一策略的优点。这些挑战包括政策与管制、消费者行为与接受度、健康、能力、科学问题和特定国家证据，以及法律、经济、农业可行性和伦理。

1 引言

根据世界卫生组织《烟草控制框架公约》第七次缔约方会议 FCTC/COP7（14）号决定 [1]，公约秘书处和世界卫生组织于 2018 年 5 月 15~16 日在德国柏林召开了一次关于降低烟草致瘾性措施的面对面会议。该会议由德国政府主办，加拿大政府协办。

会议的主要目的是评估当前和新出现的知识基础，并探讨制定和实施管制措施以降低烟草制品致瘾性的潜在好处和挑战，特别是支持或妨碍成功的条件。这些讨论构成了本报告的基础，在世界卫生组织提交第八次缔约方会议（COP8）的报告中引用，文件编号为 FCTC/COP/8/8。

会议汇集了来自世界卫生组织所有区域和一系列学科的 43 名专家①以及民间社会的代表，通过识别后果、障碍、探索国家经验和包括烟碱致瘾性的其他相关话题讨论了降低烟碱致瘾性措施的可行性、益处、风险、负面影响和机会等。会议的目的不是就所提出的任何问题达成共识，而是提出这些问题以供讨论。

---

① 与会者名单请见附录 1

2　背景文件

为确保地域和学科的多样性，世界卫生组织和 WHO FCTC 秘书处委托来自 WHO 所有区域的专家，围绕缔约方会议的要求起草八份背景文件②。

- 背景文件 1　制造潜在低致瘾性卷烟 / 烟草的可行性。
- 背景文件 2　使用潜在低致瘾性卷烟对行为的影响。
- 背景文件 3　降低烟碱 / 烟草致瘾性政策对人群和个体健康的潜在影响。
- 背景文件 4　引入潜在低致瘾性产品的监管方法和影响。
- 背景文件 5　探索除烟碱以外可导致卷烟和其他烟草制品致瘾的因素。
- 背景文件 6　探索交流与传播策略，以减少对降低烟碱或烟草致瘾性政策的误解。
- 背景文件 7　社会经济影响和向社会经济群体引入潜在低致瘾性烟草制品的后果。
- 背景文件 8　衡量降低致瘾性政策的有效性以及上市前后的监督和监测实施要求。

在会议之前，与会者收到了其他的背景文件：FCTC/COP7（14）号决定[1] 和世界卫生组织烟草制品管制研究小组（TobReg）[2] 于 2015 年发表的全球降低烟碱策略咨询说明。

---

②　本报告的附录 2~9 为这八份背景文件的概要，包括对背景文件的描述以及与会者讨论的主要内容

3 探讨降低烟草致瘾性策略

与会者审议了以下主题，讨论了关于以下方面的具体缔约方会议问题：

- 实施降低烟草致瘾性措施可能产生的积极和消极的个人和社会后果，以及成功实施降低烟草致瘾性措施的条件；
- 实施降低烟草致瘾性措施所面临的挑战；
- 任何与降低烟草致瘾性（包括烟碱成瘾）措施有关的国家经验；
- 不同群体认为应提请缔约方会议注意的其他相关事项。

3.1 假设和讨论范围

关于降低对烟草制品依赖性的讨论最初集中在可能导致烟草制品致瘾性的所有因素上，包括旨在减少或禁止某些添加剂或成分（如薄荷醇和糖）的降低潜在致瘾性措施（见背景文件5）。然而，讨论的重点是降低烟碱，特别是对燃烧型烟草制品有更多的证据。

尽管与会者没有就降低烟碱或烟草致瘾性政策的优缺点达成共识，但讨论的重点是对降低烟碱政策进行充分知情辩论的所需要素。

普遍认为，要降低对烟碱的依赖，就必须将烟草制品中烟碱的含量降低到一定水平以下。与会者认识到，正如世界卫生组织烟草制品管制研究小组（TobReg）指出的那样，导致成瘾的卷烟中的烟碱含量可能会存在产品差异 [2]。应该在技术上可行的范围内尽可能低，目前看来是每克烟丝中含有 0.4 mg 烟碱。

讨论是在假设降低烟碱政策不允许同一类别的低烟碱和常规烟碱烟草制品共存，并且可以成功实施和执行的前提下进行的。为此，强制将烟碱降至最低致瘾性水平必须是全面烟草控制方法的一部分，在该方法中成功实施关键的减少需求措施，并建立市场监督和产品测试的能力。

目前还没有可以汲取教训的降低烟草致瘾性相关的国家经验。只有美国食品药品监督管理局（FDA）发布了一份关于拟制定燃烧型卷烟中最高烟碱含量提案的预先通知。

4 实施降低烟草致瘾性措施对个人和社会潜在的积极和消极影响

关于实施旨在降低烟草制品致瘾性的降低烟碱措施对个人和社会的积极和消极影响，与会者列出了以下可能的个体影响或替代行为方式，但概率不相等且可能性未知，在整个监管背景下，可能是正面的，也可能是负面的。

4.1 对于吸烟者

（1）减少烟草制品的消费，有望促进戒烟，从而获得相关收益。

（2）吸烟者因无法合法获得高烟碱卷烟而寻求烟碱的替代来源：①在市场上使用现有的烟碱产品，如电子烟碱传输系统（EDNS）或药用烟碱；②使用其他途径获得含有烟碱的燃烧型烟草制品，如跨境购买或非法贸易，这可能会妨碍一些吸烟者完全戒烟。

4.2 对于非吸烟者

（1）受试吸烟者初始使用烟草制品的可能性降低或进展减缓。

（2）基于对降低健康风险的误解，初学者开始抽烟的可能性增加。

基于所描述的替代行为方式，人群层面的潜在后果将取决于采取不同方式的可能性。换句话说，每个吸烟者和非吸烟者都可能采取特有的行为方式，从而导致不同的人群后果，这是实验研究的主题。这类研究需要探讨各种因素，以及它们如何最大限度地发挥政策的潜在利益或积极后果，并将风险或消极后果降至最低。可能的结果在 4.3 和 4.4 节列出。

4.3　对烟草控制的预期积极社会影响

（1）吸烟的非正常化，促使局部或全球吸烟率下降。最终，吸烟率的降低将降低烟草引发的疾病发生率和死亡率。

（2）减少燃烧型烟草制品的使用，对环境有益。

（3）减少烟草相关疾病支出带来的经济效益，这将具有改善卫生的效果。

4.4　对烟草控制的假定负面社会后果

由于以下因素，吸烟率从轻微变化到增加的影响应当予以考虑。

（1）最大的担忧是烟草制品非法贸易的增加，可能导致初吸率更高，戒烟率降低，以及因非法贸易导致的低价产品的竞争和破坏烟草管制措施的其他影响使得既往吸烟者的复吸率增加。此外，它还可能影响税收，这对于政府而言是个问题。

（2）较轻一些的担忧包括：①对低致癌性产品的危害的误解可能使吸烟重新正常化，特别是对于戒烟者；②通过误导消费者这些产品和其他产品的风险或致瘾性，为烟草行业利用政策创造机会，从而妨碍政策的有效性；③烟草行业通过替代产品重塑自身；④烟草行业在实施降低烟碱政策之前游说反对烟草管制措施，推广其产品。

5 成功实施降低烟草致瘾性措施和其他与缔约方会议有关的降低烟草致瘾性事项的条件

一些与会者指出，由于缺乏一个普遍的共识，即烟碱降低策略将降低吸烟率，任何讨论成功实施的条件都为时过早。然而，人们认识到，实施降低烟碱含量从而降低烟草致瘾性措施的国家，应考虑到政策影响将取决于以下列出的某些问题以及国家监管背景。

该政策目前更适合于具有先进和全面控制措施及广泛资源和知识以确保充分实施的国家。作为一项基本先决条件，与会者注意到必须确保实施世界卫生组织《烟草控制框架公约》减少需求的关键政策措施，如与第6、8、11、13和14条有关的规定和指南。

与会者还注意到，应在一个全面的烟草控制方案的背景下评估这一政策，该方案需要一个全面的实施监管战略，并根据世界卫生组织烟草制品管制研究小组的建议确定一些先决条件。研究小组建议，"强制将烟碱减至最低致瘾性水平必须是全面烟草管制的一部分，包括增加香烟税、全面禁烟令、禁烟教育运动和图片警示标签或素包装"[2]，而且，"在缺乏成熟市场监督和产品测试能力的情况下，不建议采取降低烟草致瘾性战略。没有足够的基础设施来确保全面减少烟碱的国家应在实施这一战略之前仔细考虑提高这一方面的能力"[2]。

与会者确定了可能与缔约方会议有关或值得进一步讨论的下述内容：

- 需要认真审议和分析各国具体情况和各项措施的投资回报率，特别是对率先实施该政策的国家。尽管有大量证据表明，烟碱的降低对吸烟行为的影响比任何其他成分都大，但各国可以考虑采取较不严格的措施，包括对添加剂的管制，例如降低糖含量，这需要进一步的证据来证明它可能降低致瘾性，或消除有助于吸入的清凉剂，如薄荷醇。

- 需要一个全面的管制战略来实施、监测和执行该政策，并执行监管测试，其中包括以下内容：①全面执行世界卫生组织《烟草控制框架公约》第 9 条和第 10 条的部分实施指南。②为拟定和实施拟议政策建立足够的监管能力，并确保上市前和上市后的监督和执行。③需要从两方面思考关于降低依赖性的伦理辩论。一方面，存在与持续销售高致瘾性、高有害性烟草制品有关的伦理考虑。另一方面，对于烟碱减少措施可能带来对于高度成瘾吸烟者的挑战，也存在伦理问题。这包括考虑建立适当的支持机制，帮助吸烟者转向潜在的低风险烟碱产品或完全戒烟。④每个国家都需要一个适当的国家传播战略，目标是使决策者和普通民众反对烟草行业提出的不可行性和无效性论点。该战略应向公众传达明确的信息，阐明此类政策背后的目的和理由，以避免混淆，并预测颠覆政策的企图。⑤需要进一步培育国家特定的科学证据，以评估降低烟草致瘾性措施的适用性和潜在影响。这包括需要在国际和国家层面的监管机构之间采取协调的方法，以建立所需的证据，并根据可靠和全面的证据制定最佳做法。⑥需要充分控制非法烟草贸易。

提出的其他议题包括可能受科学共识、可行性、国家经验和国家合作影响的政策条件，以及生产足够数量的不会造成意外后果的适合烟草品种的可能性／能力，例如对农业部门（如就业）有负面影响和公共健康后果。因此，收集信息并从国家经验中吸取教训，以及促进有兴趣对燃烧型烟草制品实施降低致瘾性策略的国家之间的合作非常有意义。这种现实经验对成功实施降低烟碱政策至关重要，尽管人们认识到在现阶段许多监管问题仍未得到解决。

6 实施降低烟草致瘾性措施所面临的挑战

与会者总结了以往在国家层面实施降低烟草致瘾性政策可能面临的挑战，共包括九个方面：

（1）政策与管制挑战。例如，充分的政策支持、先行和可能失败的风险、实施时间的长短、对税收产生负面影响的风险、需要区域条约来管理新产品贸易、需要国家政策战略、偏离其他政策的风险（机会成本）和新产品的社会接受度。

（2）消费者行为与接受度挑战。例如，消费者对产品的接受程度以及制定沟通策略的需求。

（3）健康挑战。吸烟者可以尝试从其他来源获得保持他们习惯水平的烟碱，包括非法贸易的高度有害性传统烟草制品和擅自改动的产品。这可能会导致不可预见的行为影响和不可预料的市场影响，在某些情况下还会导致不可预料的健康影响。

（4）能力挑战。例如政策对适当国家战略和基础设施的要求，在机会成本[③]方面可能分散其他政策的注意力，需要向降低致瘾性产品的制造过渡过程的规则作出明确规定，总体上可能增加成本，需要能力和诀窍，以及监测能力有待增强。

（5）科学问题和特定国家证据挑战。其中包括选择降低致瘾性的方法，将研究推广至实际，定义致瘾性术语，对潜在降低致瘾性

---

③ 烟草制品管制的成本有时会被错误估计得比实际情况高。因此，机会成本计算得更加实际，且往往考虑了烟草控制的其他可能的资金来源，例如向烟草企业和制造商收取费用

产品进行分类，缺乏特定国家证据和特定产品证据。

（6）法律挑战。例如烟草行业对这一政策的反应，区域条约和贸易协定的作用，以及不断的行业创新来重塑自身。

（7）经济挑战。例如传统烟草制品非法贸易可能增加、税收可能减少、邻国之间缺乏协调和差异化的管制措施可能导致跨境非法贸易。

（8）农业可行性挑战。鉴于干预措施的复杂性和规模需要足够的生长和生产能力，这可能妨碍降低烟草致瘾性措施的及时实施。此外，这可能涉及烟草植物的基因工程（转基因生物），根据环境影响和消费者对转基因生物的认知，这可能是不同国家不同立法的主题。

（9）伦理挑战。例如，降低烟草致瘾性可能对高度成瘾的吸烟者造成影响，特别是在替代低风险烟碱产品不易获得的情况下。

7 结果和下一步计划

根据第七次缔约方会议第 FCTC/COP7（14）号决定，以面对面的会议方式讨论了目前新出现的关于降低烟草致瘾性措施的知识，主要集中缔约方会议的相关要求，即：审查对个人和社会的潜在积极和消极后果、支持成功实施的条件，以及实施的挑战。与会者注意到，关于实施该政策在全国范围内产生影响的证据有限，以及决策者需要考虑的问题非常复杂。在这一点上，与会者不希望就可能的措施达成共识，而是更愿意提醒政策制定者在审查新证据和考虑实施这一政策的可能性时应牢记潜在主题，以确保有条理和有组织的讨论。与会者还一致认为，目前不适宜在缺乏必要的国家经验的情况下制定有关烟碱降低政策的国际准则。与会者建议作者根据会议期间收到的建议审查授权论文，一旦定稿，则提交同行评审的期刊出版。

参考文献

[1] Decision FCTC/COP7(14), Conference of the Parties to the WHO Framework Convention on Tobacco Control, seventh session. Geneva: World Health Organization; 2016 (http://www.who.int/fctc/cop/cop7/FCTC_COP7(14)_EN.pdf).

[2] Advisory note: global nicotine reduction strategy: WHO Study Group on Tobacco Product Regulation. Geneva: World Health Organization; 2015.

附录1 与会者名单

Ms D. Arnott, Chief Executive, Action on Smoking and Health, London, England

Professor S. Bialous, Associate Professor in Residence, School of Nursing, University of California at San Francisco, San Francisco, United States of America (USA)

Dr K. Bromen, Key Facilitator of the WHO FCTC Article 9 and 10 Working Group, Team Leader, Tobacco Control Team, European Commission, Directorate-General on Health and Food Safety (SANTE), Unit B2 – Health in all policies, global health, tobacco control, Brussels, Belgium

Mr D. Choinière, Key Facilitator of the WHO FCTC Article 9 and 10 Working Group, Director, Tobacco Products Regulatory Office, Tobacco Control Directorate, Health Canada, Ottawa, Ontario, Canada

Mr R. Cunningham, Senior Policy Analyst, Canadian Cancer Society, Ottawa, Ontario, Canada

Professor E.C. Donny, Professor, Departments of Physiology & Pharmacology and Social Science and Health Policy, Director, Tobacco Control Center of Excellence, Wake Forest Comprehensive Cancer Center, Winston-Salem, USA

Professor M.M. Elhabiby, Associate Professor of Psychiatry, Institute of Psychiatry, Faculty of Medicine, Ain Shams University, Cairo, Egypt

Dr M. Ferech, Key Facilitator of the WHO FCTC Article 9 and 10 Working Group, Policy Officer, European Commission, Directorate-General on Health and Food Safety (SANTE), Unit B2 – Health in all Policies, Global Health, Tobacco Control, Brussels, Belgium

Ms A.M. Fernandes, Key Facilitator of the WHO FCTC Article 9 and 10 Working Group, Expert in Regulation and Health Surveillance, General Office of Tobacco and No Tobacco Products, Brazilian Health Regulatory Agency/ANVISA, Rio de Janeiro, Brazil

Professor J. Gyapong, Vice Chancellor, University of Health and Allied Sciences, Volta Region, Ghana

Mr J. Hahn, Official, Chemical and Veterinary Surveillance Institute, Sigmaringen, Germany

Professor D. Hatsukami, Forster Family Professor in Cancer Prevention, Professor of Psychiatry Associate, Director Masonic Cancer Center, University of Minnesota, Minnesota, Minneapolis, USA

Dr A. Havermans, National Institute for Public Health Environment (RIVM), Centre for Health Protection, Bilthoven, Netherlands

Dr F. Henkler-Stephani, German Federal Institute for Risk Assessment, Department of Chemical and Product Safety, Berlin, Germany

Professor V. Herrera Ballesteros, Instituto Conmemorativo Gorgas de Estudios de la Salud, Apartado, Panama

Professor S. Jhanjee, Professor of Psychiatry, National Drug Dependence Treatment Centre, WHO Collaborating Centre on Substance Abuse, All India Institute of Medical Sciences, New Delhi, India

Dr L. Bou Karroum, Researcher, American University of Beirut, Beirut,

Lebanon

Professor B. Khoorshid Riaz, Director, National Institute of Preventative and Social Medicine, Ministry of Health and Family Welfare, Dhaka, Bangladesh

Ms L.J.-e. Lee, Tobacco Control Policy Development Team, National Tobacco Control Center, Korea Health Promotion Institute, Seoul, Republic of Korea

Mr A. Luiz Oliveira da Silva, Key Facilitator of the WHO FCTC Article 9 and 10 Working Group, Specialist in Regulation and Health Surveillance, General Management of Tobacco and Non-Tobacco Products, Directorate of Authorization and Registration - DIARE, National Sanitary Surveillance Agency – ANVISA, Brasília, Brazil

Dr U. Mons, Cancer Prevention Unit, German Cancer Research Center (DKFZ), Heidelberg, Germany

Professor A.Y. Olalekan, Deputy Vice Chancellor, Research, Postgraduate Studies & Innovation, Sefako Makgatho Health Sciences University (SMU), Medunsa, South Africa

Professor L.R. Pacek, Assistant Professor, Center for Addiction Science and Technology, Department of Psychiatry & Behavioural Sciences, Duke University School of Medicine, Durham, USA

Professor G. Paraje, Senior Professor, Universidad Adolfo Ibañez, Peñalolén Santiago, Chile

Professor A. Peruga, Center for Epidemiology and Health Policies, School of Medicine/Clínica Alemana of the University del Desarrollo, Lo Barnechea, Chile (*Chair*)

Professor P.T. Phuong, Associate Professor of General Internal Medicine, Hanoi Medical University, Deputy Director of Respiratory Center, Bach Mai Hospital, Dong D, Hanoi, Viet Nam

Dr E. Pieper, German Federal Institute for Risk Assessment, Department of Chemical and Product Safety, Berlin, Germany

Dr R. Talhout , National Institute for Public Health and Environment (RIVM), Center for Health Protection, Bilthoven, Netherlands

Dr J.-P. Tassin, Directeur de Recherches Emerite Inserm, Sorbonne Université, Neuroscience Paris Seine, Paris, France

Professor R. Wittkowski, Vice President, German Federal Institute for Risk Assessment (BfR), Berlin, Germany

Professor D. Xu, Deputy Director, National Institute of Environmental Health, Chinese Center for Disease Control and Prevention, Beijing, China

WHO FCTC Secretariat

Dr V. da Costa e Silva, Head, Convention Secretariat, WHO, Geneva, Switzerland

Dr C. Audera-Lopez, Programme Manager, Convention Secretariat, WHO, Geneva, Switzerland (*Meeting coordinator*)

WHO Secretariat

Dr N.P. Cheah, Chair of the WHO Tobacco Laboratory Network, Director, Cosmetics and Cigarette Testing Laboratory, Pharmaceutical Division, Applied Sciences Group, Health Sciences Authority, Singapore

Professor G. Zaatari, Chair of the WHO Study Group on Tobacco Product Regulation, Professor & Chairman, Faculty of Medicine, The American University of Beirut, Department of Pathology and Laboratory Medicine, Beirut, Lebanon

Dr A. Blanco, Regional Advisor, Risk Factors and Nutrition, WHO Regional Office for the Americas/Pan American Health Organization, Washington, USA

Dr J. Kaur, Regional Advisor, Tobacco Free Initiative, WHO Regional Office for South-East Asia, New Delhi, India

Ms K. Lannan, Regional Advisor, Tobacco Free Initiative, WHO Regional Office for the Western Pacific, Manila, Philippines

Dr V. Prasad, Programme Manager, National Capacity, Prevention of Noncommunicable Diseases, WHO, Geneva, Switzerland

Dr R. Fayokun, Scientist, National Capacity, Tobacco Free Initiative, WHO, Geneva, Switzerland (*Rapporteur and meeting coordinator*)

Ms Miriamjoy Aryee Quansah, Prevention of Noncommunicable Diseases, WHO, Geneva, Switzerland

Dr N. Nicksic [4], Prevention of Noncommunicable Diseases, WHO, Geneva, Switzerland (*Rapporteur*)

Ms A. Vernikou [5], Prevention of Noncommunicable Diseases, WHO, Geneva, Switzerland

---

[4] An intern within the Department of Prevention of Noncommunicable Diseases from 15 March 2018 – 30 May 2018

[5] An intern within the Department of Prevention of Noncommunicable Diseases from 1 March 2018 – 30 August 2018

附录 2 背景文件 1 概要
制造潜在低致瘾性卷烟／烟草的可行性[⑥]

　　背景文件 1 探讨了制造低致瘾性烟草制品的可行性。文件讨论了有关降低烟碱的一些重要问题，如什么烟碱含量水平可以被视为非致瘾或最低致瘾，不太可能引起补偿抽吸或其他不想要的影响？其他考虑的问题包括，通过传统的农业实践、基因工程或技术改造是否可以在烟草中充分降低烟碱，以及低烟碱烟草是否能够保持足够高的吸引力，使成瘾的吸烟者自愿使用？

　　制定烟碱含量水平的标准对低烟碱卷烟的产品开发至关重要，在标准之上可能会对烟碱成瘾，但是在标准之下成瘾的可能性很小。虽然还没有确定一个明确的阈值，且应考虑到个体对烟碱的敏感性差异，但各种研究表明，将烟碱含量降低到 0.4 mg/g 可将致瘾性风险降至最低。文件概述了烟草制造商为从烟叶中去除烟碱而开发和使用的农业实践，包括基因操作和烟草制品制造技术，如超临界萃取。大多数现有技术都成功地降低了烟碱含量——基因工程和超临界萃取技术可以将烟草中的烟碱含量降低至 0.4 mg/g，但它们的有效性和可能的意外后果（如味道或某些有害物质的增加）有所不同。然而，在几乎所有情况下，由此产生的烟草都会导致不太令人满意的吸烟体验。总的来说，从技术角度来看，降低烟碱的理论是非常有科学依据且可行的。然而，卷烟的高度致瘾性也受到产品设计和制造的多种因素影响，这些因素可能为减少致瘾性提供进一步选择。

　　[⑥]　Prepared by R. Talhout, F. Henkler-Stephani, E. Pieper, A. Havermans; reviewed by H. Bozukov

尽管可以生产出烟碱含量低到足以限制其致瘾性的卷烟，但产品的用户接受度和法律问题仍有许多悬而未决的难题。通常认为影响单一和特定机制的基因修饰具有最少的非预期后果，从而产生与传统卷烟非常相似的味道。然而，基因工程在一些严格立法的国家也可能导致出现诉讼。在一些国家，监测烟碱含量是一项挑战，除烟碱之外的其他烟草添加剂可能会影响卷烟的致瘾性，如糖含量和薄荷醇。此外，对于成本影响、制造商利用烟碱的可能性以及通过所述任何技术大规模生产低烟碱烟草的时间和可行性知之甚少。

附录 3　背景文件 2 概要
使用潜在低致瘾性卷烟对行为的影响⑦

背景文件 2 考虑了引入潜在低致瘾性烟草制品的行为影响以及对市场和人群的影响。文件论述了特定目标群体的积极和消极行为影响和非预期后果、产品操作、其他烟碱来源的潜在使用以及对初吸、停止和复吸的可能影响。

降低烟碱的一个主要原因是防止青少年和年轻成年人吸烟。对于防止开始吸烟的青年人和未成年人继续吸烟，低烟碱卷烟比常规卷烟产生的促进作用要小。来自对照临床试验的数据表明，随机接受低烟碱含量卷烟的吸烟者吸烟较少，补偿性抽吸行为较低，依赖性较低，戒烟尝试和戒烟率增加。制造商可以尝试通过改变产品的成分或设计来保持卷烟的致瘾性。对烟碱减少的其他担忧与消费者的反应有关，如囤积正常烟碱含量的卷烟、篡改产品以及增加非法市场上对正常烟碱卷烟的需求。

对减少烟碱卷烟的研究表明，降低产品中的烟碱含量将降低其强化作用和致瘾性。这些变化可能会降低年轻人成为正常吸烟者的可能性，并增加当前吸烟者戒烟的可能性。目前的临床研究存在一些局限性，这些局限性可能无法代表人群或推广到其他国家，改进这些研究将建立一个降低致瘾性的证据体系。有必要开展进一步的监测研究，以评估他们的使用、停用或戒断，以及对某些群体的影响，例如对精神疾病使用者的影响和副作用。将该标准扩展到其他可有

---

⑦　Prepared by E. C. Donny; reviewed by B. Khoorshid Riaz

效替代卷烟的燃烧型烟草制品，可能对实现降低烟碱的潜在益处至关重要。已知作为卷烟行为替代品且本身具有高度有害性的产品应考虑纳入任何标准。减少卷烟和其他燃烧型产品中的烟碱可能会增加对非法产品的需求。因此，具有非燃烧替代烟碱来源的市场可能为烟碱降低策略提供更有利的条件。

附录 4 背景文件 3 概要
降低烟碱 / 烟草致瘾性政策对人群和个体健康的潜在影响⑧

背景文件 3 探讨了降低致瘾性政策对健康的潜在影响，如个体和人群水平的短期和长期健康影响。此外，该文件还讨论了对卫生服务计划的影响，包括提高认识，而不增加非预期目标群体和与培训卫生服务提供者相关的成本，且降低大多数吸烟者的总体健康风险。由于该政策没有在任何司法管辖区实施，也没有国家经验，与会者一致认为很难将健康影响作为现实数据的基础。然而，与会者建议使用良好的模型模拟以提供有关降低烟碱 / 烟草致瘾性政策对健康潜在影响的有用信息。专家们还强烈指出，这种模拟需要考虑各种环境下的可能情况，包括低收入和中等收入国家。此外，需要注意的是，根据世界卫生组织烟草制品管制研究小组的建议，个体吸烟者烟碱降低策略的最终健康效益是要求完全停止所有燃烧型烟草的使用。

---

⑧ Prepared by J. Gyapong, H. M. Mamudu, W. Agbenyikey; reviewed by P. T. Phuong

附录5 背景文件4概要 引入潜在低致瘾性产品的监管方法和影响^⑨

背景文件4探讨了实施卷烟烟碱产品标准的监管方法、实施的潜在障碍以及克服这些障碍的建议。

当降低卷烟中的烟碱含量时，与逐渐减少相比，立即减少的方法与更大、更迅速地减少烟气暴露、减少依赖和增加戒断天数有关。然而，这种方法也可能导致吸烟者更大的短期不适，这可能导致他们从其他来源寻求烟碱。可以采取一些措施来减轻卷烟中烟碱的负面影响，包括：①使用烟碱替代疗法或其他广泛使用且成本较低的药物产品。②对于一些国家，提供烟碱的其他替代来源（例如ENDS），其烟碱的有害性低于燃烧产物。③控制非法市场。全面的烟草控制（如维持或增加税收），对烟碱相关作用进行教育，通过实验室测试监测任何改变卷烟的尝试，以及监测使用率和意外后果以支持烟碱降低策略。

关于低烟碱含量卷烟的大多数研究是在美国进行的，因此研究结果对其他国家，特别是中低收入国家的普遍性是不确定的。考虑到卷烟并不总是这些国家最常用的烟草制品，有必要在美国以外开展更多的研究。需要探讨引入降低烟碱措施的实际意义，以及有关针对降低烟碱的烟草制品立法的政策关切。

由于非法市场是一个跨国问题，协调各国政策将是有益的。与实施烟碱调控（包括世界卫生组织《烟草控制框架公约》第15条的

---

⑨ Prepared by D. Hatsukami, D. Xu; reviewed by L. J-e. Lee

规定）有关的工业、农业和政府的经济负担知之甚少。此外，长期吸烟者使用低烟碱卷烟的数量以及实施这一政策的长期后果尚不清楚。值得注意的是，重点应放在减少吸烟率上，而不仅仅是减少吸烟量。

附录6 背景文件5概要 探索除烟碱以外可导致卷烟和其他烟草制品致瘾的因素[⑩]

　　背景文件5考虑了除烟碱以外的可能具有致瘾性的物质，以及可能操纵产品以影响产品致瘾性的物质。它包括对106项研究的系统综述，其中薄荷醇是研究最广泛的添加剂。所有实验性临床前研究和大多数人体研究报告了薄荷醇与致瘾性呈正相关关系。薄荷醇对戒烟行为和戒烟有不利影响，导致依赖性增强。此外，青少年、女性和非裔美国人等特定人群吸烟者对薄荷醇的依赖程度更高。

　　此外，已确认的证据表明，烟草中存在的微量生物碱，特别是在比卷烟中释放的剂量更高的情况下，可能有助于烟草制品的致瘾性。由于微量生物碱的化学结构与烟碱类似，它们的作用方式相似，但这一问题需要进一步研究。大多数烟草制品中添加了大量的糖，会在卷烟烟气中产生许多醛类化合物，如乙醛。乙醛会引发动物自我给药，可能具有致瘾性。大多数研究表明，单胺氧化酶（MAO）抑制剂增加了滥用的可能性，并可能增加低剂量烟碱的强化值。因此，这些物质在极低烟碱含量产品中的潜在作用需要进一步研究。

　　总的来说，这项系统性综述确定了支持非烟碱因素在增加烟草制品致瘾方面有潜在作用的证据。各种方法已被用于测试物质的致瘾性，但是这些方法需要标准化，并需要进一步验证。此外，还没有人群或纵向研究来确定这些因素的重要性，或它们对长期成瘾有

[⑩]　Prepared by S. Jhanjee, E. Akl, L. Bou Karroum, R. Gupta; reviewed by L. Ayo Yusuf

什么影响。确定剂量至关重要，同时也要确定烟草行业如何操纵这些因素，因为其中一些因素可能已经报告了低于影响行为的阈值剂量。此外，还需要研究了解薄荷醇以外的其他香味添加剂对烟草制品的致瘾性作用。重要的是，该文件确定了其他可能增加致瘾性的物质，并提出了哪些物质应成为监管的重点。政策可能不仅限于降低烟碱，因为这未必对每个国家都可行。

附录7 背景文件6概要 探索交流与传播策略，以减少对降低烟碱或烟草致瘾性政策的误解⑪

　　背景文件6概述了公众对烟碱和成瘾的认知，以及现有证据如何能为降低烟草制品致瘾性政策建议的一部分宣传活动提供信息。

　　围绕烟碱和成瘾的交流受到了烟草行业的影响，直到10年前烟草行业仍然否认烟碱是致瘾的，并且缺乏降低烟碱水平的举措来支持戒烟。多个国家和国际调查表明，医疗保健人员很少接受与烟草依赖治疗相关的教育，包括烟碱成瘾、戒烟和可用疗法的教育。支持减少致瘾性政策的沟通策略需要教育卫生专业人员，并在政策制定和实施的各个阶段让关键利益相关者，即消费者（吸烟者和既往吸烟者）、卫生专业人员、决策者、媒体、意见领袖参与进来。重要的是，沟通要确保将烟碱含量与烟草的整体危害分开，解决人们对低致瘾性烟草制品的误解，即误认为此类烟草制品的致癌性较小。必须进一步确保目标受众清晰，对宣传活动进行评估，并且宣传活动的投资成本是有效的。沟通策略需要政策和资源保障，对影响的评估将是关键。

　　沟通策略需要向消费者传达有关特定国家产品的信息，并确保这不是一个将促使消费者使用低致瘾性烟草制品的广告活动。确定媒体涵盖关于致瘾性和烟碱的话题，以及如何最好地导向其发展，是必要的步骤。进一步的研究可以揭示人们支持这些政策的原因，

---

⑪ Prepared by S. Bialous, B. Freeman; reviewed by D. Arnott

以及这些理由如何指导沟通策略的发展。研究还应探索政治家和决
策者的信息需求，以确保分配适当的资源，并确保在更广泛的烟草
控制措施框架内制定降低烟草致瘾性的政策。

附录8 背景文件7概要 社会经济影响和向社会经济群体引入潜在低致瘾性烟草制品的后果[12]

背景文件7回顾了社会经济群体对潜在低致瘾性烟草制品接受性差异的现有证据，以及可能的差异行为或健康影响的证据，这最终可以决定经济可行性。

当引入潜在低致瘾性烟草制品时，社会经济因素可能因为可及性/可负担性和它们对不同群体的吸烟行为或健康结果方面的差异性影响而变得很重要。分销和营销成本可能对引进这些产品的经济可行性有重要影响，特别是如果这些产品只能以高价格供应的情况下，某些群体（如低收入个人、年轻人和退休人员）会发现他们负担不起。假设满足可及性和可负担性，如果这些产品由于适口性或更好的吃味等因素对某些群体更具吸引力，且与更高的常规烟草制品戒烟率或更低的常规烟草制品初吸率有关联，则其引入将对健康结果产生直接的社会经济后果。考虑到吸烟与社会经济因素之间的联系，如贫穷或健康和教育相关支出，也有可能产生间接后果。然而，对于这些产品的市场营销的经济可行性知之甚少，因为它们在市面上非常罕见。此外，大多数临床试验都是在极低烟碱卷烟上进行的，这些卷烟有不同年龄、性别、种族的个体样本，但极少有人报告社会经济群体的不同行为。研究还表明一些群体认为烟碱与吸烟相关的癌症有关。需要提高认识以及对这些群体开展教育以消除误解。

---

[12] Prepared by G. Paraje, V. H. Herrara Ballesteros; reviewed by J-P. Tassin

确定引入具有潜在低致瘾性烟草制品的目标（例如戒烟或减少烟草抽吸量）非常重要，因为没有普遍的解决方案，应首先在全面禁烟的国家对这些产品进行研究和评估。经济问题将从不同的角度产生（例如烟草种植者、烟草企业和政府），可负担性将是一个问题。在社会经济背景下讨论税收是很重要的，因为这些产品是有害的，需要征税，但是税收应该与传统卷烟不同，而且税收应该足够高以阻止弱势群体的使用。有关使用低致瘾性烟草制品的社会经济方面的文献表明，没有足够的证据来评估在实际市场中会产生什么影响。了解在非法市场将发生什么也将是一个重要的社会经济后果。未来的研究应该包括社会经济层面的试验，这些试验可以告知决策者特定群体对引入潜在低致瘾性烟草制品会有怎样的反应。

作者指出，鉴于目前尚缺乏烟碱降低速度所带来经济后果的相关证据，因此建议采取谨慎的方法。

附录9　背景文件8概要　衡量降低致瘾性政策的有效性以及上市前后的监督和监测实施要求[⑬]

背景文件8探讨了各种短期和长期可能与评估燃烧型卷烟致瘾性降低政策有效性有关的指标。该文件还讨论了现有的机制，通过这些机制可以对每一项指标进行监督，并考虑了与这一政策相关的业务因素，包括潜在的时间表和成本。

确定了评估降低致瘾性政策有效性的措施和方法，包括烟草制品测试、烟草制品销售、烟草使用行为、烟草相关疾病的生物学指标、烟草相关的财政负担。这些指标的评估将是一项利用多种数据的重大工作，包括家庭调查、医疗保险索赔数据、基于扫描的购买行为数据。重要的是，对减少致瘾性政策的评估不应局限于评估法规目标效果的符合性（例如仅评估与燃烧型卷烟有关的使用行为）。相反，还应研究更广泛的影响（例如，评估更广泛烟草制品的相关使用行为），以及反应的非预期影响，例如烟草行业创新、产品成分或设计特性的改变，这些可能会对监管产生干扰。此外，评估这些指标的时间可能会因数据的可用性和某些指标的自然时间延长而有所不同（例如烟草相关疾病的发展）。关于实施成本，实施似乎不可避免地会产生成本。然而，这些成本可能会被收益所抵消，例如改善人群健康和降低预期的医疗支出费用。

尽管越来越多的证据表明，全国性的降低致瘾性政策将产生广

---

⑬　Prepared by L. Pacek, M. M. Elhabiby; reviewed by D. Kiptui

泛的有益影响，但一些研究问题仍未得到解答。例如，降低烟草致瘾性政策有效性的另一个指标应该包括是否出现正常烟碱含量卷烟的黑市，这是在监测研究初期应纳入的一项措施。然而，黑市的规模、性质和危害难以预测，可能与政策的实施方式、专门用于执法的资源以及含烟碱替代产品的供应有关。各国将面临不同的实施挑战，任何政策的评估都将取决于可用资源、成本与措施收益的对抗。此外，使用诸如社交媒体和短信等技术，可以有助于长期监测消费者。另一个需要监测的重要行为是寻求戒烟服务。虽然评价降低烟草致瘾性措施的有效性很重要，但尚没有一致的或国际统一的方法来评价这些措施的有效性，具体来说，没有一个适当的致瘾性降低政策最低标准要求和 / 或黄金标准。

Acknowledgements

Acknowledgements are due to all those who participated in the consultation (see Annex 1) and contributed to the development of this report by preparing background papers.

Ms Anastasia Vernikou drafted the report with support from Dr Ranti Fayokun, who coordinated the consultation process, the development of the background papers and the production of the report at WHO, under the guidance of Dr Vinayak Prasad. Professor Armando Peruga assisted with the finalization of the report. Dr Nicky Nicksic and Ms Sarah Galbraith summarized the background papers, while Dr Carmen Audera Lopez led and coordinated the consultation process at the WHO Framework Convention on Tobacco Control (WHO FCTC) Secretariat, under the leadership of Dr Vera Luiza da Costa e Silva.

Thanks also to Professor Elie Akl, Professor Hristo Bozukov, Dr Katja Bromen, Dr Nuan Ping Cheah, Mr Denis Choiniere, Mrs Priyanka Dahiya, Dr Matus Ferech, Dr Becky Freeman, Ms Marcia M Sebrao Fernandes, Dr Rishi Gupta, Ms Dorcas Kiptui, Professor Wasim Maziak, Dr Benn McGrady, Mr Andre Luiz Oliveira da Silva, Ms Moira Sy, Dr Tibor Szilagyi and Dr Ghazi Zaatari for their contributions. Ms Miriamjoy Aryee Quansah provided administrative support.

Sincere thanks are also due to the Government of Germany for hosting the consultation and providing financial, technical and administrative support, and to the Government of Canada for providing financial assistance.

Executive Summary

A meeting on tobacco addictiveness reduction measures was held in May 2018 in Berlin, Germany, as requested by the Conference of the Parties (COP) to the WHO Framework Convention on Tobacco Control (WHO FCTC).

Experts from all WHO regions discussed current and emerging knowledge on the issue and examined the potential positive and negative individual and societal consequences, as well as conditions and challenges to support successful implementation. Although there was no consensus among the participants about the merits or demerits of a nicotine or tobacco addictiveness reduction policy, discussions focused on the elements necessary for a fully informed debate, particularly of combusted tobacco products, for which more evidence is available.

Firstly, the potential individual consequences of nicotine reduction measures for smokers and non-smokers were examined. Experts deemed that the effects for smokers would include reduced consumption of tobacco products and a search for alternative sources of nicotine. However, for non-smokers, these effects would involve, on the one hand, a decreased initiation potential or decreased progression to the use of tobacco products, while on the other hand, it could lead to an increased initiation potential among novices, based on misconceptions about reduced health risk.

Additionally, experts explored the presumed societal consequences for tobacco control of a nicotine reduction strategy. Such an approach may lead to a desired denormalization of smoking, resulting in decreased smoking at local or global levels, environmental benefits due to reduced use of combusted tobacco products and economic benefits from reduced expenditure on tobacco-related diseases, which would improve health system outcomes. Conversely, the presumed negative societal consequences for tobacco control may involve an increase in illicit trade in tobacco products, possibly leading to higher initiation, decreased cessation and an increased rate of relapse by ex-smokers due to competition from low-priced products from illicit trade and other effects undermining tobacco control measures. Furthermore, it could impact on tax revenue, which could be an issue for governments.

Some experts noted that due to the lack of a consensus that a nicotine-reduction strategy would reduce smoking prevalence, any discussion of conditions for successful implementation would be premature. However, it was recognized that countries wishing to consider tobacco addictiveness reduction measures involving the lowering of nicotine content, should consider the policy impact, which will depend on national regulatory context. At the moment, this will suit countries with advanced/ comprehensive control measures and extensive resources and knowledge to ensure adequate implementation. As a fundamental prerequisite, participants noted the importance of ensuring that key demand reduction measures under the WHO FCTC, such as those contained in Articles 6, 8, 11, 13 and 14 of the Convention and their implementation guidelines adopted by the COP, be implemented. Further, mandated reductions in nicotine to minimally addictive levels must be part of a comprehensive tobacco control approach, where key demand reduction measures are successfully implemented and a developed capacity for market surveillance and product testing exists. Experts agreed that it was not opportune to develop guidelines on nicotine reduction policies at the current time, in advance of the emergence of country experience that would be valuable in informing such guidelines.

Finally, experts summarized the potential challenges to the implementation of tobacco addictiveness reduction measures under nine headings, so policy-makers can assess the merits of such a strategy in a structured manner. These are: political/regulatory, consumer acceptability, health, capacity, scientific and country specific challenges, as well as legal, economic, agricultural/ feasibility and ethical challenges.

1. Introduction

In line with decision FCTC/COP7(14) *(1)* of the seventh session of the Conference of the Parties (COP7) of the World Health Organization Framework Convention on Tobacco Control (WHO FCTC), the Convention Secretariat and WHO convened a face-to-face meeting on the theme of tobacco addictiveness reduction measures from 15–16 May 2018 in Berlin, Germany. This meeting was hosted by the Government of Germany and co-sponsored by the Government of Canada.

The main purpose was to evaluate the current and emerging knowledge base, and to explore the potential benefits and challenges of developing and implementing regulatory interventions to reduce the addictiveness of tobacco products, in particular the conditions that would support or impede success in doing so. These discussions formed the basis of this document, referenced in the WHO's report to the eighth session of the Conference of the Parties (COP8) with document number FCTC/COP/8/8.

The meeting brought together 43 experts[1] from all WHO regions and a range of disciplines, as well as representatives of civil society, to review the feasibility, benefits, risks, negative consequences, and opportunities of addictiveness reduction measures, through the identification of consequences, barriers, exploration of country experience and other

---

[1] A list of the meeting participants can be found in Annex 1.

relevant topics, including nicotine addictiveness. It was not an objective of the meeting to reach a consensus on any of the issues that were raised, but rather to map them out for discussion.

2. Background papers

WHO and the Convention Secretariat commissioned experts from all WHO regions, selected to ensure regional and disciplinary diversity, to draft eight background papers centred around the requests by the COP.[2]

- Background paper 1. Feasibility of manufacturing cigarettes/tobacco with reduced addictiveness potential.
- Background paper 2. Behavioural aspects of using cigarettes with reduced addictiveness potential.
- Background paper 3. Potential population and individual health impact of a nicotine/tobacco addictiveness reduction policy.
- Background paper 4. Regulatory approaches and implications of introducing products with reduced addictiveness potential.
- Background paper 5. Exploring factors, other than nicotine, that can contribute to the addictiveness of cigarettes and other tobacco products.
- Background paper 6. Exploring a communication/dissemination strategy to minimize misunderstanding of a nicotine or tobacco addictiveness reduction policy.
- Background paper 7. Socioeconomic consequences and consequences by socioeconomic groups of introducing tobacco products with reduced addictiveness potential.

---

2   One-page summaries of the background papers are included as Annexes 2-9 of this document. The summaries contain a description of the paper and the main comments made by the participants during discussions.

- Background paper 8. Measuring the effectiveness of an addictiveness reduction policy, pre/post market surveillance and monitoring requirements for implementation.

Prior to the meeting, participants received additional background documents: Decision FCTC/COP7(14) *(1)* and the Advisory Note on Global Nicotine Reduction Strategy by the WHO Study Group on Tobacco Product Regulation (TobReg) *(2)* published by WHO in 2015.

3. Discussion on the tobacco addictiveness reduction strategy

Participants considered the following topics, addressing specific COP questions on:

- the potential positive and negative individual and societal consequences of implementing tobacco addictiveness reduction measures, as well as the conditions that would support the successful implementation of tobacco addictiveness reduction measures;
- the challenges to implementation of tobacco addictiveness reduction measures;
- any relevant country experience associated with tobacco addictiveness reduction measures, including nicotine addictiveness; and
- any other related matter that in the opinion of this diverse group should be brought to the attention of COP.

3.1 Assumptions and scope of discussions

The discussion on the reduction of dependence on tobacco products focused initially on all factors that could contribute to the addictiveness of all tobacco products, including potential dependence reduction measures aimed at reducing or banning certain additives or constituents, such as menthol and sugars (see background paper 5). However, discussions focussed on nicotine reduction, particularly of combusted tobacco products, for which more evidence is available.

Although there was no consensus among participants about the merits or demerits of a nicotine or tobacco addictiveness reduction policy, discussions focused on the elements necessary for a fully informed debate on a nicotine reduction policy.

It was considered that to achieve a reduction of dependence on nicotine entails the reduction of nicotine content in tobacco products below a certain level. Participants recognized that the nicotine content of cigarettes that leads to dependence is likely to vary individually as noted by the WHO Study Group on Tobacco Product Regulation (WHO TobReg) *(2)*. This should be as low as is technically feasible and currently would appear to be 0.4 mg nicotine per gram of cigarette tobacco filler.

The discussion proceeded under the assumption that a nicotine reduction policy would not allow coexistence of reduced nicotine and regular nicotine tobacco products within the same category and would require successful implementation and enforcement. To do so, mandated reductions in nicotine to minimally addictive levels must be part of comprehensive tobacco control approach where key demand reduction measures are successfully implemented and a developed capacity for market surveillance and product testing exists.

There is currently no country experience from which to derive lessons in reducing tobacco addictiveness. Only the United States Food and Drug Administration (FDA) has issued an advanced notice of proposed rule-making to implement a rule on the maximum level of nicotine in combusted cigarettes.

4. Potential positive and negative individual and societal consequences of implementing tobacco addictiveness measures

In deliberating the positive and negative individual and societal consequences of implementing the use of reduced nicotine tobacco product measures designed to reduce addiction to tobacco products, participants mapped out the following individual responses or alternative behavioural paths that are possible, but of unequal and sometimes unknown probability, and which may be positive or negative depending on the regulatory context.

4.1 For smokers

1. Reduced consumption of tobacco products, hopefully leading to cessation and therefore obtaining its associated gains.
2. Seeking alternative sources of nicotine because smokers would not be able to legally obtain high nicotine cigarettes:
   i. use of available nicotine products in the market, such as Electronic Nicotine Delivery Systems (ENDS) or medicinal sources of nicotine;
   ii. use of combusted tobacco products containing nicotine from alternative sources, such as cross-border purchases or the illicit trade, which could prevent some smokers from completely quitting.

4.2 For non-smokers

1. Decreased initiation potential or decreased progression to the use of

tobacco products for experimental smokers.

2. Increased initiation potential by novices, based on misconceptions about reduced health risk.

Based on the alternative behavioural paths described, the potential consequences at population level would depend on the likelihood of the different paths. In other words, the likelihood that each individual smoker and non-smoker may adopt specific behavioural paths and therefore lead to different population consequences is a subject for empirical studies. Such research would need to explore the various factors and how they could maximize the policy's potential benefits or positive consequences and minimize the risks or negative consequences. Possible outcomes include those listed below.

4.3 Presumed positive societal consequences for tobacco control

1. Denormalization of smoking, leading to decreased smoking at local or global levels. Ultimately the reduction of smoking prevalence would reduce mortality and morbidity from tobacco-attributable diseases and conditions.
2. Some environmental benefits due to reduced use of combusted tobacco products.
3. Economic benefits from reduced expenditure on tobacco related diseases, which would improve health system outcomes.

4.4 Presumed negative societal consequences for tobacco control

Consideration should be given to effects ranging from insignificant smoking prevalence changes to its increase due to the factors below.

1. A primary concern is an increased illicit trade in tobacco products, possibly leading to higher initiation, decreased cessation and an increased relapse by ex-smokers due to competition from low-priced products from illicit trade and other effects undermining tobacco control measures. Furthermore, it could impact on tax revenue, which is an issue for governments.

2. Less likely concerns, include:

    i. misconceptions about the harm of reduced addictiveness products and possible renormalization of smoking, especially for those who have quit;

    ii. creating opportunities for the tobacco industry to exploit the policy by misleading consumers about the risk or addictiveness of these and other products, and thus preventing the possible effectiveness of the policy;

    iii. the tobacco industry reinventing itself through alternative products; and

    iv. the tobacco industry lobbying against tobacco control measures in general and promoting its products in advance of the implementation of the reduced nicotine policy.

5. Conditions that would support successful implementation of tobacco addictiveness reduction measures and other tobacco addictiveness reduction-related matters relevant to COP

Some participants noted that due to the lack of a general consensus that a nicotine-reduction strategy would reduce smoking prevalence, any discussion of conditions for successful implementation would be premature. However, it was recognized that countries considering implementation of tobacco addictiveness reduction measures involving the reduction of nicotine content, should take into account that policy impact will depend on the certain issues set out below as well as the national regulatory context.

The policy is more suited at the moment to countries with advanced/comprehensive control measures and extensive resources and knowledge to ensure adequate implementation. As a fundamental prerequisite, participants noted the importance of ensuring that key WHO FCTC policy measures to reduce demand, such as provisions and guidelines in relation to Articles 6, 8, 11, 13 and 14, be implemented.

Participants also noted that such a policy should be assessed within the context of a comprehensive tobacco control programme, requiring a comprehensive regulatory strategy for implementation, with certain preconditions in line with the recommendations of the WHO Study Group on Tobacco Product Regulation. The study group recommended that "mandated reductions in nicotine to minimally addictive levels in cigarettes must be part of comprehensive tobacco control, including increased taxes on cigarettes, comprehensive smoking bans, anti-smoking educational campaigns and graphic warning labels or plain packaging", *(2)* and that, "a strategy to reduce the addictiveness of tobacco is not recommended in the absence of developed capacity for market surveillance and product testing. Countries without adequate infrastructure to ensure a comprehensive approach to nicotine reduction should carefully consider increasing that capacity before implementing such a strategy" *(2)*.

The (study group) participants identified the following which might be relevant to the COP, or merit further discussion

- The need for careful deliberation and analysis of the country-specific situation and return-on-investment of various measures, particularly for countries initially implementing the policy in isolation. Although there is substantially more evidence that nicotine reduction will have an effect on smoking behaviour than for any other constituent, countries could consider less stringent measures, including the regulation of additives, for example a reduction of sugar, which requires further evidence of its possible impact on dependence reduction or elimination of cooling agents like menthol, which facilitate inhalation.
- The need for a comprehensive regulatory strategy to implement, monitor and enforce such a policy and to perform regulatory testing, which would include the following.
  - Full implementation of the partial guidelines on Articles 9 and 10 of the WHO FCTC.
  - Building adequate regulatory capacity for the development and implementation of the proposed policy and ensuring pre- and post-market surveillance and enforcement.

– The need to ponder both sides of the ethical debate on reduction of dependence. On the one hand, there are ethical considerations related to the persistent sale of highly addictive, highly toxic tobacco products. On the other hand, there are ethical issues with regards to the challenges that nicotine reduction measures would pose to highly addicted smokers. This includes contemplating the institution of suitable support mechanisms to assist smokers wanting to switch to potentially lower-risk nicotine products or full cessation.

– The need for a suitable national communication strategy in each country aimed at both policy-makers and the general population to counter the tobacco industry's non-feasibility and non-effectiveness argument. The strategy should have clear messages to the public which articulate the purpose and rationale behind such a policy to avoid confusion, and to anticipate attempts to subvert the policy.

– The need to foster further country-specific scientific evidence to assess the suitability and potential impact of tobacco addictiveness reduction measures. This includes the need for a coordinated approach amongst regulators at international and national levels to build the required evidence and formulate best practice based on reliable and robust evidence.

– The need for adequate control of the illicit tobacco trade.

Other topics raised included political conditions which could be influenced by the scientific consensus, feasibility, country experience and country cooperation, and the possibility/ability to produce suitable tobacco strains in sufficient quantities and in a manner that will prevent unintended consequences, such as a negative impact on the agricultural sector (for example employment) and public health consequences.

Therefore, it is relevant to gather information and learn from country experience(s), as well as to promote collaboration among countries with an interest in implementing a strategy to reduce the dependence from combusted tobacco products. Such real-life experience could be crucial to the successful implementation of a nicotine reduction policy, although it is recognized that many regulatory questions remain unanswered at this stage.

6. The challenges to implementation of tobacco addictiveness reduction measures

Participants summarized the previous discussion on the potential challenges to the implementation of a tobacco addictiveness reduction policy at country level under nine headings.

1. Political/regulatory challenges – such as adequate political support, risk of going first and possibly failing, length of time for implementation, risk of a negative impact on tax revenue, need for regional treaties to regulate trade of new products, need of country strategy for policy, risk of distraction from other policies (opportunity costs) and social acceptance of new products.

2. Behavioural/acceptability challenges – such as consumer acceptance of products and the need to develop a communication strategy.

3. Health challenges – smokers could try to maintain the same levels of nicotine which they are accustomed to getting from other sources, including illicitly traded highly toxic conventional tobacco products and tampered products. This may lead to unforeseen behavioural implications, unanticipated market effects, and in some cases, unexpected health effects.

4. Capacity challenges – such as the requirements for a suitable country strategy and infrastructure for the policy, potential for distraction from other policies in terms of opportunity costs,[3] the need for clarity over

---

3 The cost of tobacco product regulation is sometimes wrongly assumed to be higher than it really is. Therefore, opportunity costs should be calculated realistically and always consider potential additional sources of funding from tobacco control, such as charging costs to tobacco companies or manufacturers.

the rules governing the process of transitioning to manufacturing of addictiveness reduction products, potential increased costs in general, need for capacity and know-how, and lack of monitoring capacity.

5. Scientific and country specific evidence challenges – which include the choice of approach to reducing addictiveness, translation of research into real life, the definition of the addictiveness term, classification of products with reduced addictiveness potential, lack of country-specific evidence and lack of product specific evidence.

6. Legal challenges – such as the response of the tobacco industry to such a policy, the role of regional treaties and trade agreements, constant industry innovation to reinvent itself.

7. Economic challenges – such as the potential increase of illicit trade of conventional tobacco products, possible decrease in tax revenue, lack of coordination and differentiated regulatory treatment between neighbouring countries which may lead to cross-border illicit trade.

8. Agricultural/feasibility challenges – given the complexity and magnitude of intervention requiring adequate growing and production capacity, which could impede the timely implementation of tobacco addictiveness reduction measures. Furthermore, this may involve genetic engineering of tobacco plants which may be the subject of differing legislation in different countries, in the light of the environmental impact and consumer perception of genetically modified organisms (GMOs).

9. Ethical challenges – such as the possible impact on highly addicted smokers affected by tobacco addictiveness reduction, particularly if alternative lower-risk nicotine products were not readily available.

7. Outputs and next steps

As requested by COP7 and in accordance with COP Decision FCTC/ COP7(14), current and emerging knowledge on tobacco addictiveness reduction measures were discussed at a face-to-face meeting, which focused primarily on the COP request to examine the potential positive and negative individual and societal consequences, the conditions to support successful implementation, and the challenges to implementation. Participants noted the limited evidence on the countrywide effects of implementing the policy and the complexity of the issues to be considered by policy-makers. At this point, rather than trying to reach a consensus on possible measures, participants preferred to map out the potential topics that policy-makers should bear in mind to ensure a methodical and structured discussion when reviewing new evidence and contemplating the possibility of implementing such a policy. Participants also agreed that it was not opportune to develop international guidelines on the nicotine reduction policy at the current time, in advance of the necessary country experience that would be valuable in informing such guidelines.

Participants proposed that authors review the commissioned papers according to the recommendations received during the meeting and once finalized, submit them to a peer-reviewed journal for publication.

References

1. Decision FCTC/COP7(14), Conference of the Parties to the WHO Framework Convention on Tobacco Control, seventh session. Geneva: World Health Organization; 2016 (http://www.who.int/fctc/cop/cop7/FCTC_COP7(14)_EN.pdf).
2. Advisory note: global nicotine reduction strategy: WHO Study Group on Tobacco Product Regulation. Geneva: World Health Organization; 2015.

Annex 1.   List of participants

Ms D. Arnott, Chief Executive, Action on Smoking and Health, London, England

Professor S. Bialous, Associate Professor in Residence, School of Nursing, University of California at San Francisco, San Francisco, United States of America (USA)

Dr K. Bromen, Key Facilitator of the WHO FCTC Article 9 and 10 Working Group, Team Leader, Tobacco Control Team, European Commission, Directorate-General on Health and Food Safety (SANTE), Unit B2 – Health in all policies, global health, tobacco control, Brussels, Belgium

Mr D. Choinière, Key Facilitator of the WHO FCTC Article 9 and 10 Working Group, Director, Tobacco Products Regulatory Office, Tobacco Control Directorate, Health Canada, Ottawa, Ontario, Canada

Mr R. Cunningham, Senior Policy Analyst, Canadian Cancer Society, Ottawa, Ontario, Canada

Professor E.C. Donny, Professor, Departments of Physiology & Pharmacology and Social Science and Health Policy, Director, Tobacco Control Center of Excellence, Wake Forest Comprehensive Cancer Center, Winston-Salem, USA

Professor M.M. Elhabiby, Associate Professor of Psychiatry, Institute of Psychiatry, Faculty of Medicine, Ain Shams University, Cairo, Egypt

Dr M. Ferech, Key Facilitator of the WHO FCTC Article 9 and 10 Working Group, Policy Officer, European Commission, Directorate-General on Health and Food Safety (SANTE), Unit B2 – Health in all Policies, Global Health, Tobacco Control, Brussels, Belgium

Ms A.M. Fernandes, Key Facilitator of the WHO FCTC Article 9 and 10 Working Group, Expert in Regulation and Health Surveillance, General Office of Tobacco and No Tobacco Products, Brazilian Health Regulatory Agency/ANVISA, Rio de Janeiro, Brazil

Professor J. Gyapong, Vice Chancellor, University of Health and Allied Sciences, Volta Region, Ghana

Mr J. Hahn, Official, Chemical and Veterinary Surveillance Institute, Sigmaringen, Germany

Professor D. Hatsukami, Forster Family Professor in Cancer Prevention, Professor of Psychiatry Associate, Director Masonic Cancer Center, University of Minnesota, Minnesota, Minneapolis, USA

Dr A. Havermans, National Institute for Public Health Environment (RIVM), Centre for Health Protection, Bilthoven, Netherlands

Dr F. Henkler-Stephani, German Federal Institute for Risk Assessment, Department of Chemical and Product Safety, Berlin, Germany

Professor V. Herrera Ballesteros, Instituto Conmemorativo Gorgas de Estudios de la Salud, Apartado, Panama

Professor S. Jhanjee, Professor of Psychiatry, National Drug Dependence Treatment Centre, WHO Collaborating Centre on Substance Abuse, All India Institute of Medical Sciences, New Delhi, India

Dr L. Bou Karroum, Researcher, American University of Beirut, Beirut,

Lebanon

Professor B. Khoorshid Riaz, Director, National Institute of Preventative and Social Medicine, Ministry of Health and Family Welfare, Dhaka, Bangladesh

Ms L.J.-e. Lee, Tobacco Control Policy Development Team, National Tobacco Control Center, Korea Health Promotion Institute, Seoul, Republic of Korea

Mr A. Luiz Oliveira da Silva, Key Facilitator of the WHO FCTC Article 9 and 10 Working Group, Specialist in Regulation and Health Surveillance, General Management of Tobacco and Non-Tobacco Products, Directorate of Authorization and Registration – DIARE, National Sanitary Surveillance Agency – ANVISA, Brasília, Brazil

Dr U. Mons, Cancer Prevention Unit, German Cancer Research Center (DKFZ), Heidelberg, Germany

Professor A.Y. Olalekan, Deputy Vice Chancellor, Research, Postgraduate Studies & Innovation, Sefako Makgatho Health Sciences University (SMU), Medunsa, South Africa

Professor L.R. Pacek, Assistant Professor, Center for Addiction Science and Technology, Department of Psychiatry & Behavioural Sciences, Duke University School of Medicine, Durham, USA

Professor G. Paraje, Senior Professor, Universidad Adolfo Ibañez, Peñalolén Santiago, Chile

Professor A. Peruga, Center for Epidemiology and Health Policies, School of Medicine/Clínica Alemana of the University del Desarrollo, Lo Barnechea, Chile (*Chair*)

Professor P.T. Phuong, Associate Professor of General Internal Medicine,

Hanoi Medical University, Deputy Director of Respiratory Center, Bach Mai Hospital, Dong D, Hanoi, Viet Nam

Dr E. Pieper, German Federal Institute for Risk Assessment, Department of Chemical and Product Safety, Berlin, Germany

Dr R. Talhout , National Institute for Public Health and Environment (RIVM), Center for Health Protection, Bilthoven, Netherlands

Dr J.-P. Tassin, Directeur de Recherches Emerite Inserm, Sorbonne Université, Neuroscience Paris Seine, Paris, France

Professor R. Wittkowski, Vice President, German Federal Institute for Risk Assessment (BfR), Berlin, Germany

Professor D. Xu, Deputy Director, National Institute of Environmental Health, Chinese Center for Disease Control and Prevention, Beijing, China

WHO FCTC Secretariat

Dr V. da Costa e Silva, Head, Convention Secretariat, WHO, Geneva, Switzerland

Dr C. Audera-Lopez, Programme Manager, Convention Secretariat, WHO, Geneva, Switzerland (*Meeting coordinator*)

WHO Secretariat

Dr N.P. Cheah, Chair of the WHO Tobacco Laboratory Network, Director, Cosmetics and Cigarette Testing Laboratory, Pharmaceutical Division, Applied Sciences Group, Health Sciences Authority, Singapore

Professor G. Zaatari, Chair of the WHO Study Group on Tobacco Product Regulation, Professor & Chairman, Faculty of Medicine, The American University of Beirut, Department of Pathology and Laboratory Medicine, Beirut, Lebanon

Dr A. Blanco, Regional Advisor, Risk Factors and Nutrition, WHO Regional Office for the Americas/Pan American Health Organization, Washington, USA

Dr J. Kaur, Regional Advisor, Tobacco Free Initiative, WHO Regional Office for South-East Asia, New Delhi, India

Ms K. Lannan, Regional Advisor, Tobacco Free Initiative, WHO Regional Office for the Western Pacific, Manila, Philippines

Dr V. Prasad, Programme Manager, National Capacity, Prevention of Noncommunicable Diseases, WHO, Geneva, Switzerland

Dr R. Fayokun, Scientist, National Capacity, Tobacco Free Initiative, WHO, Geneva, Switzerland (*Rapporteur and meeting coordinator*)

Ms Miriamjoy Aryee Quansah, Prevention of Noncommunicable Diseases, WHO, Geneva, Switzerland

Dr N. Nicksic,[4] Prevention of Noncommunicable Diseases, WHO, Geneva, Switzerland (*Rapporteur*)

Ms A. Vernikou,[5] Prevention of Noncommunicable Diseases, WHO, Geneva, Switzerland

---

4   An intern within the Department of Prevention of Noncommunicable Diseases from 15 March 2018 – 30 May 2018.

5   An intern within the Department of Prevention of Noncommunicable Diseases from 1 March 2018 – 30 August 2018.

Annex 2.   Summary of background paper 1 – Feasibility of manufacturing cigarettes/tobacco with reduced addictiveness potential[6]

Background paper 1 explores the feasibility of manufacturing less addictive tobacco products. The paper addresses some important questions on nicotine reduction, such as what level of nicotine can be regarded as non- or minimally addictive and is unlikely to provoke compensatory smoking or other undesired effects. Other questions considered include whether it is feasible to reduce nicotine sufficiently in tobacco either by traditional agricultural practice, genetic engineering or by technical modifications, and whether low or reduced nicotine free tobacco can maintain a sufficiently high appeal to be voluntarily used by addicted smokers.

Setting standards for the levels of nicotine above which addiction is likely and below which addiction is less likely is vital in the development of reduced nicotine cigarettes. Although a clear threshold has not been defined yet and individual differences in sensitivity to nicotine should be accounted for, various studies indicate that decreasing nicotine content to 0.4 mg/g would minimize the risk for dependence. This article provides an overview of agricultural practices, including genetic manipulation, and tobacco product manufacturing techniques, such as supercritical extraction, that have been developed and used by tobacco manufacturers to remove nicotine from tobacco leaves. Most of the available techniques are successful in reducing nicotine levels – genetic

---

6   Prepared by R. Talhout, F. Henkler-Stephani, E. Pieper, A. Havermans; reviewed by H. Bozukov.

manipulation and superficial extraction can reduce nicotine levels to 0.4 mg/g in tobacco – but differ in their effectiveness and their possible unintended consequences e.g. flavour or increased amounts of certain toxicants. However, in almost all cases the resulting tobacco leads to a less satisfactory smoking experience. In general, the rationales to reduce nicotine are very well founded and feasible from a technical perspective. However, the high dependence potential of cigarettes is also affected by multiple factors of product design and manufacture that might provide further options to reduce addictiveness.

Even though producing cigarettes with nicotine levels low enough to limit addiction is possible, there are many unanswered questions concerning user acceptability of the product and legal issues. Genetic modifications that affect single and specific mechanisms are generally thought to have the fewest unintended consequences, thus resulting in a flavour quite similar to regular cigarettes. However, genetic modification may also lead to issues in countries with strict legislation. Monitoring nicotine levels can be challenging in some countries, and other tobacco additives besides nicotine may influence addictiveness of cigarettes, such as sugar levels and menthol. Furthermore, little is known about the cost implications, possibilities for exploitation by manufacturers, and timing and feasibility of large-scale production of reduced nicotine tobacco by any of the techniques described.

Annex 3.   Summary of background paper 2 – Behavioural aspects of using cigarettes with reduced addictiveness potential[7]

Background paper 2 considers the behavioural implications and the impact on the market and population of introducing tobacco products with reduced addictiveness potential. The paper addresses positive and negative behavioural implications and unintended consequences among specific target groups, manipulation of products, potential use of other sources of nicotine, and the possible effects on initiation, cessation and relapse.

A central reason for reducing nicotine is to prevent youth and young adults from becoming smokers. To prevent continued use among youth and minors who initiate smoking, reduced nicotine cigarettes should produce fewer positive effects than regular conventional cigarettes. Data from controlled clinical trials show that smokers randomized to receive cigarettes low in nicotine smoked fewer cigarettes, had low compensatory smoking behaviour,

were less dependent and had an increase in quit attempts and abstinence from smoking. However, a potentially important unintended consequence of reducing nicotine is that consumers could perceive low nicotine products as safer. Manufacturers could attempt to maintain the addictiveness of cigarettes by altering the content or design of the product. Other concerns about nicotine reduction relate to consumer responses such as hoarding

---

7   Prepared by E. C. Donny; reviewed by B. Khoorshid Riaz.

of normal nicotine content cigarettes, product tampering, and increased demand for illicit market normal nicotine cigarettes.

Studies of reduced nicotine cigarettes suggest that reducing the level of nicotine in the product will render it less reinforcing and less addictive. These changes may both decrease the probability that naïve youth will become regular smokers and increase the probability that current smokers will quit. There are limitations in current clinical studies that may not be representative of the population or generalizable to other countries, and improving these studies will build a body of evidence for reducing addictiveness. Future surveillance studies are necessary to assess their use, cessation/withdrawal, and effects on certain groups, such as dosing and side effects for those with psychiatric conditions. Extending the standard to other combusted tobacco products that effectively substitute for cigarettes may be critical to realizing the potential benefits of nicotine reduction. Products that are known to function as behavioural substitutes for cigarettes and are highly toxic themselves, should be considered for inclusion in any standard. Reducing nicotine in cigarettes and other combusted products may increase demand for illicit products. Consequently, markets with non-combusted alternative sources of nicotine may provide more favourable conditions for a nicotine reduction strategy.

Annex 4.   Summary of background paper 3 – Potential population and individual health impact of nicotine/ tobacco addictiveness reduction policy[8]

Background paper 3 explores potential health impact of an addictiveness reduction policy, such as short- and long-term health impact at the individual and population levels. Additionally, this paper addresses the implications on health services programmes, including raising awareness without promotion to unintended target groups and costs associated with training health service providers, and the potential reduction in the overall health risks of most smokers. As the policy has not been introduced in any jurisdiction and there is no country experience, participants agreed that it would be difficult to base health impact on real life data. However, the use of good simulation models which could provide useful information on the possible health impact of a nicotine/tobacco addictiveness reduction policy was suggested in the meeting. Experts also strongly stated that such simulations will need to consider possible scenarios in various settings including low- and middle-income countries. Further, it is to be noted that as recommended by the WHO Study Group on Tobacco Product Regulation, the ultimate health benefits of a nicotine reduction strategy for individual smokers will require complete cessation of intake of all combusted tobacco.

---

8   Prepared by J. Gyapong, H. M. Mamudu, W. Agbenyikey; reviewed by P. T. Phuong.

Annex 5. Summary of background paper 4 – Regulatory approaches and implications of introducing products with reduced addictiveness potential[9]

Background paper 4 examines the regulatory approaches to implementing a nicotine product standard for cigarettes, potential barriers for implementation, and recommendations to overcome these barriers.

When lowering the level of nicotine in cigarettes, an immediate reduction approach is associated with a greater and more rapid overall reduction in smoke exposure, decrease in dependence and a higher number of abstinence days compared to gradual reduction. However, this approach may also lead to greater short-term discomfort among smokers, which would potentially lead them to seek nicotine from other sources. Several measures can be implemented to mitigate any negative impact from reducing nicotine in cigarettes, which include: i) making access to nicotine replacement therapies or other widely available and less costly pharmacological products; ii) for some countries, providing other alternative sources of nicotine, which are less toxic than combusted products (e.g., ENDS); and iii) controlling illicit markets. Comprehensive tobacco control (e.g. maintaining or increasing taxes), education about the effects of nicotine, laboratory testing to monitor any attempts to alter cigarettes, and surveillance to determine prevalence of use and monitor unintended consequences would support a nicotine reduction approach.

The majority of the studies on reduced nicotine content cigarettes

---

9   Prepared by D. Hatsukami, D. Xu; reviewed by L. J-e. Lee.

have been conducted in the United States of America, therefore the generalizability of the study results to other countries, particularly in middle- and low-income countries, are uncertain. More studies outside of the United States of America are necessary, considering that cigarettes are not always the most used tobacco products in these countries. The practical implications of introducing nicotine reduction measures need to be explored, as well as political concerns about legislation on tobacco products targeted for nicotine reduction.

As the illicit market is a problem across borders, coordinating policy across countries would be beneficial. Relatively little is known about the economic burden for industry, farmers and governments associated with the implementation of nicotine regulation, including the provisions of Article 15 of the WHO FCTC. Additionally, how long-term smokers will use reduced nicotine cigarettes and the long-term consequences of implementing this policy are unknown. It is important to note that the focus should be on reducing smoking prevalence and not only the number of cigarettes smoked.

Annex 6.   Summary of background paper 5 – Exploring factors, other than nicotine, that can contribute to the addictiveness of cigarettes and other tobacco products[10]

Background paper 5 considers substances other than nicotine that might have addictiveness properties and potential manipulation of products to influence product addictiveness. It includes a systematic review of 106 studies, where menthol was the most widely studied additive. All experimental pre-clinical studies and most human studies reported a positive association between menthol and addictiveness. Menthol adversely impacts quitting behaviour and tobacco cessation, leading to increased dependence potential. Further, higher dependence levels amongst menthol smokers were found in certain subgroups such as adolescents, women, and African-Americans.

Additionally, the identified evidence suggests that minor alkaloids present in tobacco, particularly at doses higher than delivered in cigarettes, could possibly contribute to some of the dependence potential of tobacco products. As the chemical structure of alkaloids is similar to nicotine, they act in a similar way, but the issue requires further research. Sugars added in high quantities to most tobacco products give rise to numerous aldehydes, such as acetaldehyde, in tobacco smoke. Acetaldehyde is self-administered by animals and is potentially addictive. Most studies suggested that monoamine oxidase (MAO) inhibitors increased abuse liability and may increase the reinforcing value of low doses of nicotine. Thus, the potential role of these substances in very low nicotine content

---

10   Prepared by S. Jhanjee, E. Akl, L. Bou Karroum, R. Gupta; reviewed by L. Ayo Yusuf.

products will require further research.

Overall, this systematic review identified evidence supporting the potential role of non-nicotinic factors in increasing the dependence potential of tobacco products. However, varied methods for testing the addictiveness of substances have been used which need standardization and require further validation. Also, there are no human or longitudinal studies to determine the importance of these factors, or what impact they will have in addictiveness long-term. Determining dose is critical, as well as determining how the tobacco industry can manipulate these factors, as some of these factors could have reported doses that are below the threshold that affects behaviour. Additionally, there is a need to undertake research on understanding the roles of flavour additives other than menthol for their contribution to the addictiveness of tobacco products. Importantly, this paper determines other substances that could increase addictiveness and raises questions on what substance should be the focus for regulation. Policy may not be limited to nicotine reduction only as it may not be feasible for every country.

Annex 7.   Summary of background paper 6 – Exploring a communication/ dissemination strategy to minimize misunderstanding of a nicotine or tobacco addictiveness reduction policy[11]

Background paper 6 provides an overview of what is known about the public's perception of nicotine and addiction, and how available evidence could inform a communications campaign adopted as part of a tobacco products addictiveness reduction policy recommendation.

Communication surrounding nicotine and addiction has been influenced by both the tobacco industry, which until a decade ago denied that nicotine was addictive, and the lack of initiatives promoting lower levels of nicotine as a strategy to support quitting. Multiple national and international surveys have shown that healthcare professionals receive little-to-no education related to tobacco dependence treatment, including education on nicotine addictiveness, withdrawal and available therapies. A communication strategy to support an addictiveness reduction policy would need to educate health professionals and involve key stakeholders – consumers (i.e. smokers and ex-smokers), health professionals, policy-makers, media, opinion leaders – in all stages of policy development and implementation. Importantly, communication would ensure that the message uncouples overall tobacco harm from nicotine content and addresses the misperception that reduced addictiveness tobacco products are less carcinogenic. It would further have to ensure that the target

---

11   Prepared by S. Bialous, B. Freeman; reviewed by D. Arnott.

audience is clear, the campaign is evaluated, and that investments on communications campaign are cost effective. A communication strategy requires political and resources commitment, and an evaluation to assess impact will be key.

A communication strategy needs to convey information about country-specific products to consumers and ensure that it is not an advertising campaign that would drive consumers to use reduced addictiveness tobacco products. Identifying media coverage on the topic of addictiveness and nicotine, and how best to influence it going forward, are necessary steps. Future research could shed light on the reasons why people support these policies and how such rationale could guide the communication strategy development. Research should also explore the informational needs of politicians and policy-makers to ensure that proper resources are allocated and that any policy to reduce the addictiveness of tobacco occurs within a broader framework of tobacco control measures.

Annex 8.   Summary of background paper 7 – Socioeconomic consequences and consequences by socioeconomic groups of introducing tobacco products with reduced addictiveness potential[12]

Background paper 7 reviews the existing evidence on differential acceptability of tobacco products with reduced addictiveness potential by socioeconomic groups and the evidence on differential behaviours or health effects they may have, which could ultimately determine economic feasibility.

When introducing tobacco products with reduced addictiveness potential, socioeconomic factors can be important due to the accessibility/ affordability and the differential impact they may have in terms of smoking behaviour or health outcomes on different groups. Distribution and marketing costs may have an important influence on the economic viability of the introduction of these products, especially if they are only available at high prices, in which case certain groups (e.g., low-income individuals, young and retired people) will find them inaccessible. Given accessibility and affordability, if these products are more appealing to some groups due to factors such as palatability or better smell and they are linked to, for instance, higher probabilities of quitting regular tobacco products or a lower probability of initiation of regular tobacco product consumption, their introduction will have direct socioeconomic consequences on health outcomes. It is also possible that indirect consequences will be present, given the link between smoking and

---

12   Prepared by G. Paraje, V. H. Herrara Ballesteros; reviewed by J-P. Tassin.

socioeconomic factors, such as poverty or health and education-related expenditures. However, little is known about the economic feasibility of marketing these products, as they have rarely been marketed. Further, most clinical trials have been conducted on very low nicotine cigarettes and these have samples of individuals of different ages, sex, ethnicities, with very few of them reporting differential behaviours by socioeconomic group. Studies have also shown that some groups believe that nicotine is related to smoking-related cancers. Such misconceptions will need to be addressed by raising awareness and running educational campaigns to educate these groups.

Determining the goal (e.g. cessation or reduction of tobacco) of introducing tobacco products with reduced addictiveness potential would be important since there will not be a universal solution, and research and evaluation of these products should be performed in countries with comprehensive tobacco bans first. Economic issues would exist from different perspectives (e.g. tobacco growers versus tobacco industry versus government), and affordability would be an issue. Discussing taxation would be important in the socioeconomic context, as these products are harmful and need to be taxed, yet taxation should vary from relative to conventional cigarettes and be high enough to discourage use among vulnerable groups. The description of the literature found on socioeconomic aspects related to the use of reduced addictiveness tobacco products shows that there is not enough evidence to assess what would be the impact in an actual market. Understanding what will happen in the illicit market will be an important socioeconomic consequence as well. Future research should include experiments and trials on socio-economic dimensions that could inform policy-makers about how specific groups would react to the introduction of tobacco products with reduced addictiveness potential.

The authors indicated that given that there is no evidence of the economic consequences of the speed at which nicotine reduction should be introduced and recommended a cautious approach.

Annex 9. Summary of background paper 8 – Measuring the effectiveness of an addictiveness reduction policy, pre/post market surveillance, and monitoring requirements for implementation[13]

Background paper 8 explores various short- and long-term indicators that may be relevant to evaluating the effectiveness of an addictiveness reduction policy for combusted cigarettes. This paper also discussed the existing mechanisms by which each of these indicators may be surveilled and operational considerations, including the potential timelines and cost implications, associated with such a policy.

Measures and methods were identified to evaluate the effectiveness of an addictiveness reduction policy, including: tobacco product testing; tobacco product sales; tobacco use behaviours; biological indicators of tobacco-related disease; and tobacco-related financial burden. Evaluation of these indicators will be a large undertaking utilizing many types of data, including household surveys, health insurance claims data, scanner-based purchasing behaviour data. Importantly, evaluations of an addictiveness reduction policy should not be limited to assessing compliance within the intended effects of a regulation (e.g. only evaluating use behaviours related to combusted cigarettes). Rather, they should also study the broader effects (e.g. evaluating use behaviours related to a wider spectrum of tobacco products), as well as unintended effects of responses, such as tobacco industry innovation, manipulation of product content or design features,

---

13   Prepared by L. Pacek, M. M. Elhabiby; reviewed by D. Kiptui.

that may interfere with the impact of regulation. Additionally, timelines for evaluating these indicators are likely to vary based on availability of the data and a prolonged natural time course for some indicators to manifest (e.g. development of tobacco-related diseases). Regarding cost implications, it is likely unavoidable that implementation will incur costs. However, these costs may be offset by the benefits, such as improved population health and anticipated healthcare expenditure savings.

Despite an accumulating evidence base suggesting that a nationwide addictiveness reduction policy would have broad beneficial effects, a number of research questions remain unanswered. For example, an additional indicator of effectiveness of an addictiveness reduction policy could include the emergence of a black market for normal nicotine content cigarettes, a measure needed for inclusion at baseline of surveillance studies. However, the size, nature, and harm of the black market are difficult to predict and would likely be related to how the policy is implemented, the resources dedicated to enforcement and the availability of alternative nicotine containing products. There will be implementation challenges that differ by country and evaluation of any policy will depend on resources available and the costs versus the benefits of the measure. Additionally, the use of technology, such as social media and texting, could be useful to monitor consumers over time. Another important behavioural aspect to monitor is access to cessation services. Whilst it would be important to evaluate the effectiveness of tobacco addictiveness reduction measures, there is no consensus or internationally agreed approaches to evaluate the effectiveness of such measures, specifically if there is an adequate minimum standard required and or a gold standard for an addictiveness reduction policy.